HAIR CARE BASICS THAT SAVE MONEY

HAIR CARE BASICS THAT SAVE MONEY

DEBORAH ROSS
AND
ARLON BEAUREGARD

iUniverse LLC
Bloomington

HAIR CARE BASICS THAT SAVE MONEY

iUniverse books may be ordered through booksellers or by contacting:

iUniverse LLC
1663 Liberty Drive
Bloomington, IN 47403
www.iuniverse.com
1-800-Authors (1-800-288-4677)

ISBN: 978-1-4759-9469-8 (sc)
ISBN: 978-1-4759-9470-4 (ebk)

Printed in the United States of America

iUniverse rev. date: 07/16/2013

We dedicate this book to all cancer survivors and
to the families of those who lost the battle.

We acknowledge and appreciate Aaron Westmoreland and
Stephanie Minus for their assistance in completion of our book.

A Special Thank you, to Rachel Quinn Photography
rayequinnphotography.com

CONTENTS

CHAPTER 1

Definition of Hair

Hair is composed of a protein called *keratin*, which is the same protein found in our nails and in our skin. Hair contains *melanin,* which determines the color of the hair.

A strand of hair has three layers. The outermost layer is called the cuticle. It is transparent and its function is to protect the inner layers. The innermost layer is called the medulla and is composed of large, loose cells that may have a hollow-like appearance. Between these two layers is the cortex.

Hair grows from the follicle (a pocket in the skin). This saclike structure surrounds the root of the hair and is found beneath the skin. Tiny blood vessels provide nutrition. During the growing phase the bottom is shaped like a bulb. The papilla (inside the bulb) is fed by tiny blood vessels that bring in oxygen and food and take away waste products. The papilla is sensitive to hormones and the chemicals (medicines) secreted by our bodies. This process may slow or increase growth, or the hair may not grow at all because of the amounts of hormones or chemicals secreted.

The color, shape, and thickness of your hair is basically determined by genetics. Take a look at your parents and grandparents!

We have approximately 150,000 hairs on our heads and typically lose 50–100 hairs per day.

Hair Types

It is beneficial to know as much as you can about your hair type prior to purchasing hair products. It will not only save you money, but buying the appropriate product will improve and enhance the health and beauty of your hair. For example, if your hair is dry and brittle, you would want products that repair the damage rather than products that further dry out your hair. Knowledge of your hair type will also help you select hairstyles that work best for you.

Determine your hair type by identifying which of the following four hair types is yours:

1) Straight Hair—Hair appears straight to the ends and may be difficult to curl, perm, or style.
2) Wavy Hair—When the hair is wet, it forms into a loose S-shape. It is easier than straight hair to style, which can be accomplished by allowing hair to dry naturally, eliminating the need to use heat on the hair. The hair texture may range from fine to coarse.
3) Curly Hair—Curly hair has tighter S-shaped curls as the hair dries. It may be difficult to manage and may require a permanent (relaxer) or a reverse permanent to loosen the curls and allow the hair to be styled, especially if the hair is coarse.
4) Kinky Hair—Kinky hair has the most defined curl type, appearing like a zigzag and being tightly coiled; this hair type is less S-shaped and more Z-shaped. This type of hair is the most fragile and requires a delicate hand when drying, combing, brushing, or exposing it to heat, as it is prone to breakage/damage.

Hair Textures

Hair texture is determined by the width of the hair strand and can be described as fine, medium, or coarse. Knowing your type of hair texture allows you to select and purchase hair products specific to the needs of your hair.

Fine Hair: Fine hair is small in diameter and almost weightless and has a tendency to "fly away." If it is straight, it has difficulty holding a curl. Fine hair usually takes to chemical processing easily, but caution must be used when applying perms, relaxers, and other chemicals because it is easy to overprocess this type of hair.

Medium Hair: Medium hair is better known as "normal" hair. If your hair is not fine, flyaway, coarse, or thick, it is considered medium texture. Medium hair is the easiest to manage and the easiest to process. Hair with medium texture usually takes perms and relaxers well.

Coarse Hair: The texture of coarse hair is considered the strongest, as the diameter of the hair is thick—even feeling rough to the touch. Thick, coarse hair can be difficult to manage and style, so a perm or relaxer may be required to soften and make the hair more manageable.

Problems—Hair

Many people experience hair and/or scalp problems. The hair may become thin or brittle, break off, or fall out. Itching, flaking, or scaling of the scalp can cause scalp discomfort. These conditions may or may not be associated with a serious or chronic medical condition.

Hair Thinning and/or Hair Loss

Protein is the leading factor in physical growth. It also regulates and maintains hair. Your hair is composed of approximately 86 percent protein (keratin), which protects the hair. When hair protein is broken down, your hair becomes dry, brittle, and damaged.

Protein deficiency can contribute to hair thinning and loss, but it takes a long time for protein deficiency to become apparent, as the body will use stored protein from muscle and tissue before signs are visible. A lack of protein in your diet can cause brittle nails, hair thinning, split ends, or hair loss. The use of protein supplements will help increase protein levels if you are not eating the recommended daily requirement.

A client once came into the salon complaining about how thin her hair had become. At the age of ninety, her appetite was poor, which often occurs in the senior population. I explained the importance of protein in her diet and encouraged her to eat foods or supplements high in protein. She added peanut butter, cheese, and nuts to her diet to increase her protein intake. We also used a Nioxin treatment weekly, and after six to eight weeks, new hair growth began to appear.

Warning: With chronic protein deficiency, changes in activity levels (tired, low energy) and lowered heart rate (less than 60 bpm) will become apparent. If you are experiencing extreme hair loss or any of these conditions, consult a physician for a medical evaluation.

Causes of Hair Thinning or Loss

- ✓ alopecia
- ✓ sudden physical and/or emotional stress
- ✓ pregnancy or delivery (hormonal changes)
- ✓ high fever
- ✓ severe infections
- ✓ major surgery
- ✓ low-protein crash dieting
- ✓ thyroid conditions
- ✓ sudden blood loss
- ✓ anemia
- ✓ lupus
- ✓ syphilis
- ✓ radiation or chemotherapy
- ✓ medications, such as:
  - o birth control pills
  - o beta blockers
  - o calcium channel blockers
  - o NSAIDS
- ✓ continuous use of hair extensions

Hair loss caused by menopause or childbirth usually returns to normal after six to twenty-four months. Hair loss caused by illnesses, radiation, or chemotherapy usually grows back on its own. Although hair treatments are not required in these cases, they can help slow hair loss and restore hair to a healthier condition.

As an example, a dear friend of mine was undergoing chemotherapy, and she began to lose large amounts of hair. I suggested that she get a short haircut, replace her shampoo and conditioner with Nioxin Treatment System, and apply an additional protein deep-conditioning treatment weekly. After a few weeks, her hair loss began to slow down. Both treatments were continued during and after chemotherapy, and in the end she retained about half of her original hair, and the new growth came back thick and healthy. There is no guarantee this approach would work for everyone, but it worked for her.

Problems—Scalp

The condition of the scalp has a lot to do with the health and appearance of the hair. Fungal infections cause flaking, itching, or crusting of the scalp, so an extremely dry, flaky scalp may be a sign of a medical condition. A client of mine had a dry, flaky scalp that did not respond to normal dandruff treatments over a period of time, so I suggested she consult a doctor, who diagnosed her with diabetes. The signals our bodies give us that something is wrong are amazing!

Problems of the Scalp

- ✓ acne or pimples
- ✓ eczema (itchy, swelling or redness of the skin)
- ✓ sunburn (can lead to cancer of the skin)
- ✓ infections and rashes caused by HIV
- ✓ psoriasis or seborrhea
- ✓ folliculitis (infection or inflammation of the hair follicle)
- ✓ head lice (tiny insects)
- ✓ ringworm (circular rash patch on scalp)

When to Contact a Medical Professional

- Hair loss is in an unusual pattern, such as females with male-patterned baldness or males with other patterns of baldness.
- Hair loss is rapid or occurs in the teens or twenties.
- Hair loss is accompanied by pain or itching.
- There is excessive flaking of the scalp.
- There is acne on the scalp.
- Women grow unusual amounts of facial hair.
- There are scaly, red areas on the scalp.
- There are bald spots in the beard or eyebrows.
- Hair loss is accompanied by weight gain, muscle weakness, intolerance to cold temperatures, or fatigue.

You might want to consult this site for additional information regarding scalp conditions: http://www.webmd.com.

CHAPTER 2

Hair Products

Shampoos

First things first! If you are getting ready to shampoo in the shower, don't make the common mistake of forgetting the shampoo and thinking that using a bar of soap or liquid body soap will do the same job. Bath soaps are made to clean the body, not the hair. Bath soaps can cause hair damage and breakage and can give hair a dull appearance. When selecting your shampoo, try to avoid shampoos that contain alcohol, which dries out the hair. Most stores carry numerous types of shampoos:

- ✓ shampoos for normal hair
- ✓ gentle shampoos for oily hair
- ✓ moisturizing shampoos for dry/brittle hair
- ✓ protein-based shampoos for damaged hair
- ✓ shampoos for color-treated hair
- ✓ shampoos that build hair body for fine, limp hair

Conditioners

There are multiple types of hair-conditioning products:

Protein Packs: Protein packs are thick and heavy and contain a high amount of surfactants that help bind hair structure. Protein packs are left in the hair for longer than most conditioners, and some require heat application to assist in hair penetration. Because of chemical reactions, protein packs have high viscosity and tend to form thick layers on the hair.

Leave-in Conditioners: Leave-in conditioners have a thinner consistency and different surfactants and chemical makeup than protein packs. The product is lighter and less viscous and forms a thinner layer on the hair.

Regular Conditioners: Regular conditioners can be either leave-in or package conditioners. They are used after shampooing the hair, and users often choose the same product name as the shampoo used.

Moisturizers: Moisturizers hold moisture in the hair and usually contain high proportions of humectants, whose function is to retain moisture in the hair. In very dry air, hair can become frizzy, unruly, or flyaway. In tropical climates with high humidity, curly hair, if it is dry and damaged, absorbs moisture from the air, causing it to swell and be frizzy. The hair feels rough and can become tangled, leading to hair breakage.

Reconstructors: Reconstructors usually contain hydrolyzed protein, whose function is to penetrate the hair and strengthen its structure.

Acidifiers: Acidifiers regulate hair acidity by maintaining the conditioner's pH around 3.5.

Thermal Protectors: Thermal protectors are heat-absorbing polymers that help protect the hair against excessive heat caused by blow-drying, hot rollers, curling irons, and flat irons.

Glossers: Glossers are light-reflecting chemicals that bind to the hair surface (polymers).

Oils: Oils are usually EFAs—essential fatty acids—which can help dry/porous hair to become more soft and pliable. The scalp produces a natural oil called sebum, and EFA oil is the closest oil to natural sebum. (Sebum contains EFA oil.)

Humectants: Humectants are used in skin and hair products to promote moisture retention. These hygroscopic compounds create a chemical structure that attracts water from the atmosphere and binds it to various sites along the hair molecule.

How to Choose Hair Products

So many hair products are on the market that it is difficult to decide which to use, and not all products are right for your hair type or condition. At one time professional hair products had to be purchased at a hair salon, but today they are available at drug stores and grocery stores. The following information will help you select the right products for your hair type and condition—the ones that are best for *your* hair.

Fine Hair: If you have fine or flyaway hair, choose shampoos and conditioners with labels that include words like "featherweight," "volumizing," "for fine hair," or "for thin hair." These products will add volume and help maintain your style. The use of antihumidity products is a must if you live in a humid tropical climate. Choose styling products that include words like "ultra-light," "volumizing," and "for fine, limp hair."

Wavy Hair: For wavy hair, select shampoo and conditioners that are for "normal to dry hair" and creamy shampoos and conditioners with "moisturizers." If you use heat to style your hair, use smoothing lotions, thermal lotions, creams, and gels to get the results you want.

Curly Hair: Curly hair requires hair products that are creamy and contain moisturizers. Purchase products that are "hydrating" and that contain antihumidity agents. Styling products with an oil base, such as finishing crèmes, smoothing lotions, wrap lotions, or thermal lotions, will give the best styling results. For curly, frizzy hair use frizz-control hair products.

Coarse Hair: Hydrating shampoos and conditioners are what you need, as these products contain moisturizers for dry, brittle hair. Styling products with an oil base, such as crèmes, wrap lotions, and smoothing and thermal lotions, will help give you the hairstyle you want. If your hair is coarse and frizzy, additional hair care should include protein packs that contain oil, replenishing hair masks, or products for frizz control.

Hair Care Equipment

The number-one cause of hair damage is heat. It is extremely important to select the correct equipment and heat setting for your hair type.

The key to a good hairstyle is using a wall-mounted, pull-out mirror. A pull-out mirror is a necessary tool to keep your hands free for cutting or styling your own hair.

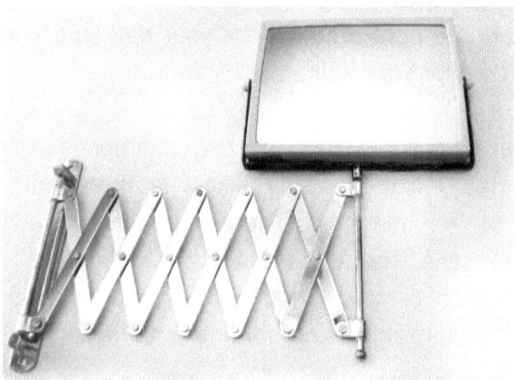

Blow-Dryers

Blow-Dryer Safety: Before using your blow-dryer, read the manufacturer's warnings and instructions, including any instructions in or on the box and the safety label on the cord of the hair dryer. Check your plug periodically for frayed wiring before using your blow-dryer.

There are several types of blow-dryers to choose from that will allow you to own the equipment that fits your hair type and texture:

Ionic dryers minimize frizz and lock in moisture and shine.

Ceramic dryers eliminate hot spots, have plenty of power, and do not overheat.

Tourmaline dryers boost ionic power in order to reduce drying time.

Infrared dryers reduce drying time by half, which results in less hair damage.

Several blow-dryer attachments and features are available:

Diffusers can be used on fine, color-treated, permed, or naturally curly hair. They work by diffusing heat so the hair dries slowly at a cooler temperature.

Air-flow concentrators are the opposite of diffusers, as they narrow the end of the blow-dryer and concentrate the air to a small area, speeding drying time.

Comb nozzles work like concentrators but have a built-in comb.

Cool-shot buttons are used to finish and hold your style. First use the heat button to remove moisture, and then continue your style with a brush, using the cool-shot button to complete your style.

Be sure to select the correct wattage for your hair type and texture.

For *fine and damaged hair*, use 1200 to 1500 watts.

For *thick, wavy hair*, use 1800 to 1875 watts.

For *thick, coarse hair*, start at 2000 watts.

Flat Irons

There are several types of flat irons to choose from:

Ceramic iron plates disperse heat evenly for fast, safe styling. Ceramic irons lock in moisture and leave hair shiny and smooth.

Tourmaline iron plates balance hair and reduce static electricity and frizz.

Ionic iron plates balance hair to eliminate static electricity and frizz, add shine, and cause hair to feel softer.

Titanium iron plates are smooth and give snag-free styling.

Infrared flat irons with tourmaline, titanium, ceramic, and infrared technology recondition and reconstruct your hair while maintaining healthy hair.

What to Purchase for Your Hair Type and Texture

Suggested shopping list (temperatures vary by product).

Fine or Thin Hair

    short length—½–1¼-inch plate
    shoulder length—1–1½-inch plate
    long length—1¼–2-inch plate
    temperature—below 360° F

Normal or Wavy Hair

    short length—½–1¼-inch plate
    shoulder length—1–1½-inch plate
    long length—1¼–2-inch plate
    temperature—360–380° F

Thick, Coarse, or Curly Hair

    short hair—1–1½-inch plate
    shoulder-length hair—1–2-inch plate
    long hair—1½–2-inch plate
    temperature—380–410° F

Curling Irons

Purchasing the right curling iron for your hair is key. Curling iron barrels come in several widths and types of material. The wider the width, the looser your curls will be. The materials used include ceramic and tourmaline in addition to the usual metal. Curling irons also come in several styles, including spring, clipless, marcel, brush, spiral, and double and triple barrel. Follow the label and safety instructions.

Benefits of Ceramic and Tourmaline

- ✓ heats quickly
- ✓ eliminates static electricity
- ✓ neutralizes odor
- ✓ preserves moisture in the hair shaft
- ✓ causes less damage

Heat Settings for Your Hair Type

- ✓ Fine, fragile, or chemically treated hair: start at 200–250° F
- ✓ Normal, curly, or thick hair: start at 280–300° F
- ✓ Thick, coarse, curly hair: start at 300–400° F

Some irons have settings above 400°, so use caution; start at 300° and gradually increase the temperature until you reach the desired curl, as you don't want to burn your hair and leave the curl on the curling iron. Make sure you work with hair that is relatively straight and dry, and use a heat-protecting product.

Haircutting Equipment

comb
sharp scissors
clippers with attachments
wall-mounted (pull-out) mirror so you can see the back of your head

Equipment for Perms

rat-tailed comb
perm rods of various sizes
large hair clips to section the hair
wall-mounted (pull-out) mirror

Equipment for Hair Relaxers

chemical brush
rat-tailed comb
large-tooth comb
large clips to section the hair
wall-mounted (pull-out) mirror

CHAPTER 3

Shampooing and Conditioning

Some think it isn't important to know the type of shampoo and conditioner their hair needs to maintain hair health and beauty or how often to shampoo. The following information will be helpful in keeping your hair healthy and ensuring you can have good-looking hairstyles.

We shampoo our hair to clean it and to promote and maintain hair health. Shampoo removes dirt and oil buildup from the hair. If your hair is extremely oily or begins to smell sour easily, daily shampooing may be indicated, while dry to normal hair may require shampooing only once or twice per week.

It is important to shampoo your hair two to three days prior to applying any chemical to your hair, such as a relaxer. I once had a client who decided to relax her hair at home, but she failed to use shampoo and condition her hair regularly and had not done so in a month. As a result, she lost hair in large patches shortly after relaxing her hair. When she came to my salon for help, I applied an ApHogee treatment system, followed by a protein deep conditioner. Fortunately, the hair loss decreased after the first treatment. At that point I cut her hair into a shorter style that allowed her to wear a natural look. It took approximately six weeks for hair breakage to stop completely and evidence of restoration and new growth to appear. Depending on the extent of the damage, the recovery time may vary.

Proper Method for Applying Shampoo

1. Select the appropriate shampoo for your hair type.
2. Wet hair thoroughly.

3. Apply shampoo the size of a quarter into the palm of the hand.
4. Work the shampoo through the hair to loosen and remove dirt until all hair is covered with shampoo.
5. Rinse hair thoroughly.
6. Apply shampoo a second time, repeating the instructions above. If your hair has a good amount of lather, your hair is clean. If not, repeat the shampoo instructions until the hair shampoo lathers.
7. Rinse hair thoroughly.
8. Gently squeeze the water from your hair.
9. Gently blot—do not rub—hair with a towel.*

*Rubbing the hair can cause split ends.

Why Condition?

This step restores moisture, shine, and luster to the hair. If your hair is curly or coarse, use a leave-in conditioner after you have blotted your hair dry.

Proper Method for Applying a Conditioner

1. Select the appropriate conditioner for your hair type.
2. Apply a quarter-sized amount into the palm of your hand.
3. Work the conditioner through your hair.
4. With a large-tooth comb, comb the conditioner through your hair.
5. Wait three to five minutes.
6. Rinse the hair until it is clear of conditioner.
7. Gently blot—do not rub—the hair with a towel.*

*Rubbing the hair dry with a towel can cause split ends.

Deep Conditioning

Deep-conditioning treatments are useful when the hair is dry or damaged and requires additional protein and oils. These treatments can be purchased from beauty supply stores, which carry good selections of a variety of deep conditioners and hair-repair therapies.

1. Shampoo the hair first.
2. Apply the deep conditioner generously to the hair.
3. Massage it into the scalp using your fingertips.
4. Comb through with large-tooth comb.
5. Put on a plastic cap.
6. Sit under a dryer for ten to fifteen minutes.
7. Remove cap and rinse hair until clear.

Shampoo without Shampoo!

Place a nylon stocking over a stiff-bristle hairbrush and brush the hair thoroughly to remove dirt, flakes, and styling products. It works well as a temporary fix when water or time is limited. Waterless shampoos are available at beauty supply and medical supply stores.

How to Stimulate Hair Growth

Massage the scalp with the balls of your fingertips for three to five minutes to increase blood flow to the surface of the scalp, which feeds the hair follicles that promote hair growth. You can also use a pulsating shower attachment when rinsing your hair in the shower to stimulate hair growth.

Hair-stimulating products are available at beauty salons and beauty supply stores.

A Tip for Swimmers

Apply leave-in conditioner to the palm of your hand and work the conditioner into the hair before getting into the water. After swimming, shampoo with clarifying shampoo, which can lift hair color (make it lighter). Apply leave-in conditioner after swimming.

Antistatic Tips

Use deep conditioners regularly, as moisturized hair is less likely to be affected by static. You can also use an antistatic spray on your hairbrush, and leave-in hair conditioners or conditioning hair gels help reduce static. Run a fabric softener dryer sheet over your hair as needed to reduce static. Avoid using hair products that contain alcohol, which will dry your hair out.

Deep-Conditioning Treatment Recipe for Dry or Damaged Hair

½ cup mayonnaise
2 tablespoons olive oil
$1/8$ teaspoon soy sauce

Mix the ingredients together. Apply the mixture by working it through the entire head, and comb it through. Place a plastic cap on the head and leave it on for fifteen to twenty minutes. Natural body heat will help the treatment penetrate the hair. Rinse the hair, and apply shampoo if needed (if hair is too oily).

Hot-Oil Treatment

Work three tablespoons of olive oil (may substitute with jojoba, coconut, or sunflower oil) into the hair. Place a plastic cap over the hair and sit under a hair dryer for ten to fifteen minutes. If you don't have a dryer, leave the cap on for thirty to forty-five minutes, using your natural body heat. Shampoo, rinse, and condition your hair.

Tip: Foods rich in omega-3 fats are beneficial to hair health, and drinking six to eight glasses of water per day will help keep your hair and skin hydrated.

Hairstyle Techniques

Blow-Drying Hair 101

Before using a blow-dryer or any thermal equipment, blot your hair with a towel to remove as much water as possible. Apply a heat-protecting styling product, work it through the hair with your fingers, and then comb it through with a large-tooth comb.

Step 1:

> At this point the hair should be slightly damp (not wet). You can also let it dry naturally until it is damp or use a vent brush on cool to medium heat until the hair is slightly damp. Your fingers moving through the hair will accomplish the same results as the vent brush while blow-drying the hair. Separate the hair into five sections, leaving the nape (above the neck) area loose.

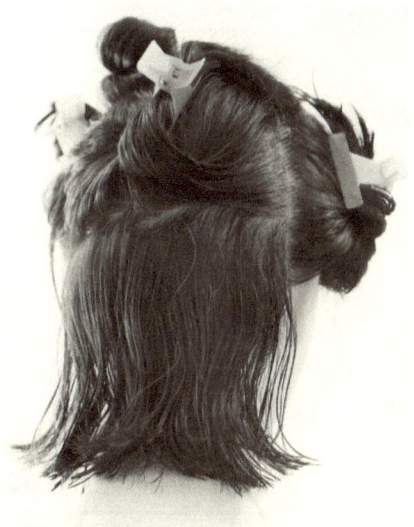

Step 2:

Take the hair from the nape area, and starting near the scalp with a round bristle brush placed under a small section of the hair, pull the hair downward while wrapping hair around the brush. You can also turn the hair upward into a "flip" by placing the brush on top and wrapping the hair strands upward around the brush while pulling the brush toward the end of the hair.

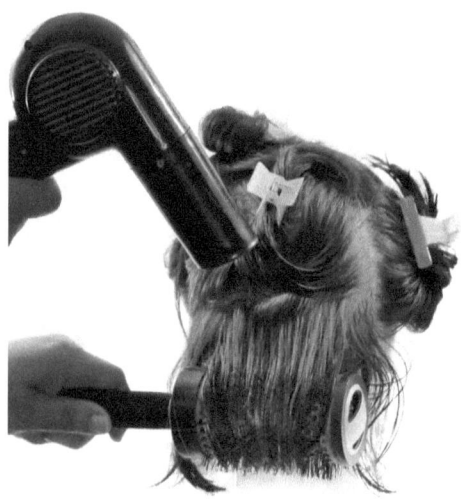

Step 3:

Complete one side of the sectioned hair at a time in the same fashion, working up toward the top of your head. After both sides are complete, finish the top of the hair. Allow the hair to cool before combing or brushing it into the desired style. Apply a finishing spray if desired to hold your hairstyle.

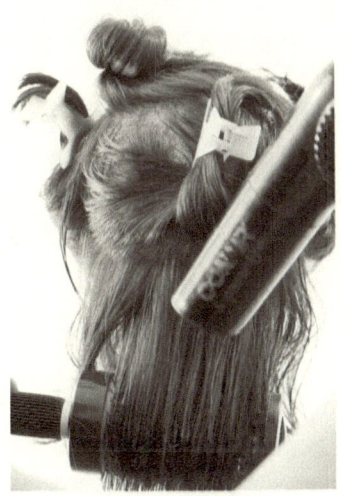

Finished blow-dry style

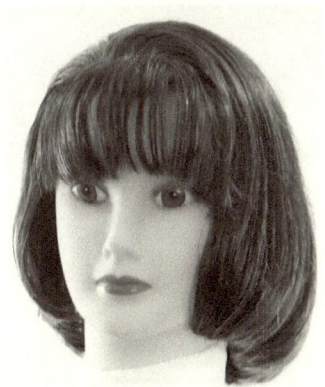

How to Blow-Dry Curly Hair and Maintain a Curly Style

Whether you have naturally curly hair or your hair has been permed, the blow-drying process is the same.

Step 1:

> Blot the hair with a towel to remove excess water. Apply a styling gel or crème to the damp hair, working it in from the roots to the ends.

Step 2:

> Attach a diffuser to the blow-dryer, and turn it on at the low speed. (The diffuser attachment on the blow-dryer controls the flow of air on the hair.) Cup a section of the hair in your hand, holding it loosely, and pull it away from the head. Hold the dryer above your head at a ninety-degree angle to give volume to the hair as you dry. Dry one section at a time until the entire head is dry. Apply a sheen and finishing product. To complete the style use a pick or wide-tooth comb.

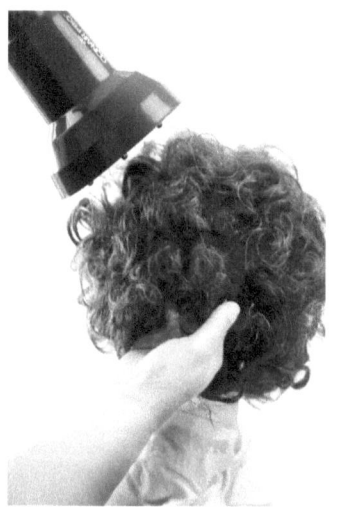

How to Blow-Dry Long Hair

Flip your head forward so the hair flows over your face, and dry with the diffuser for a minute or two to add volume.

Curly-Hair Tip

> Twist one small section of hair at a time with the fingers. Use a diffuser on low to medium heat, and follow the instructions for blow-drying curly hair. Finish the style with a sheen product or finishing spray if desired.

Styling with a Curling Iron

The size of the curl will be determined by the size of the curling iron barrel. Choose a size that will give you the style desired—small, medium, or large curls.

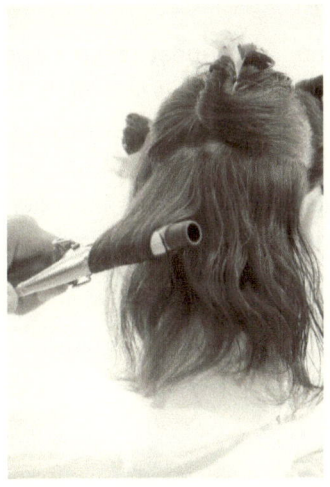

Step 1:

> Preheat the curling iron. Apply a heat-protecting product to the palm of your hand and work the product through the hair.

Step 2:

> Let your hair naturally dry or use a blow-dryer or hooded dryer. (Follow previous blow-drying instructions.) The hair should be completely dry prior to using the curling iron. (If you attempt to

dry the hair with the curling iron, you will burn your scalp with the steam and heat and cause hair damage from the heat.)

Step 3:

Separate the hair into five sections, leaving nape area (above the neck) loose. Starting at the nape area, take a section of hair ½–1 inch wide and clamp the ends between the barrel of the curling iron and its holder (the top part that clamps onto the barrel). Make sure no hair shows on the other side of the holder. Slowly turn the iron under to curl the hair, and continue rolling under until you are near the scalp. Hold for ten seconds and release.

Slide the curl off the iron with a comb, and repeat these steps until you have the desired number of curls. Allow the curls to cool, and then brush or comb the curls into the desired style.

To avoid getting the curling iron tangled in the hair, as this often happens, keep hair in the middle of the barrel and away from the handle.

Use a finishing spray or hair sheen product as desired.

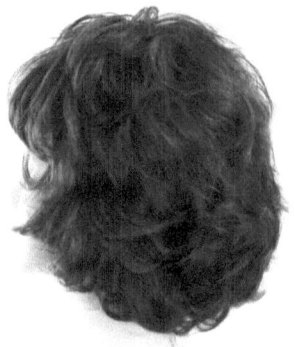

Flat Iron

The same method as that for a curling iron is used for styling with a flat iron, with one exception, as the flat iron is not used to roll the hair under to the scalp area. Dry your hair completely from the tips to the roots. Use a straightening balm on your hair after it has been dried, which will eliminate frizz and protect your hair. Application of a heat-protective spray to your hair will help defend your hair against damage caused by heat-based styling tools like flat irons.

Use the flat iron on approximately two-inch segments of the hair at a time. Place the flat iron close to, but not touching, the scalp and move it in a continuous downward motion toward the end of the hair. Repeat these steps until the desired amount of hair is straightened. Hair ends may be left straight, turned up, or turned under. Complete the style with finishing spray as desired.

Roller Setting

There are many types of hair rollers available. Hot rollers, Velcro rollers, and magnetic rollers are a few of the most commonly used types.

Hot-Roller Tip: Prior to using hot rollers, apply a styling product. Blow-dry the hair straight, and then follow the rolling instructions below.

Velcro or Magnetic-Roller Tip: When using Velcro or magnetic rollers, leave the hair damp for best results. Then apply a styling product and follow rolling instructions listed below.

Step 1:

> Part the hair to the desired style. Take a small section of hair (to fit the roller) and wrap it around the roller 1½–2 times. (The size of the curl depends on the roller size: tight curl = small roller, loose curl = large to extra-large roller). For hard-to-wrap hair, use end papers, which help keep straight hair from sticking out while you are wrapping the hair.

Step 2:

> To complete the application of rollers, first roll the front hair, then both sides of the head, and finish with the back of the head. Now you are ready to dry your hair, which can be accomplished by drying hair naturally or by sitting under a hooded or cap dryer for forty to sixty minutes.

Step 3:

> Once the hair is completely dry, allow the hair to cool for a few minutes. Then remove the rollers and comb or brush the hair into the desired style. Finally, apply a finishing spray.

How to Trim Hair with Scissors

Have you ever gone to a salon and had a bad haircut? Here are tips to help you get the desired style and haircut when you go to the salon.

Why Do I Need to Know about Haircuts If I Am Going to a Salon?

Good communication with the stylist will help you achieve the cut and style you are looking for! For example, if you go to a salon and tell the stylist you want a layered cut, you need to know the difference between a short layered cut and a long layered cut. If you want long layers, you may want to have the stylist cut only a few inches off your hair. If you want short layers, the stylist may have to cut off more than a few inches to get the desired style and cut. It would be a shame to end up with a short layered cut when you really wanted a long layered hairstyle.

Cutting Tips for All Hair Types

Fine Hair: A blunt cut (hair cut straight across) will make your hair appear thicker; a body wave will give your hair a similar appearance.

Straight Hair: When your hair is straight, a soft, angled, layered cut (cut on an angle or slant) will soften the hair's appearance and add texture and movement to your hair. A body wave before the haircut will soften the hair and improve its flexibility.

Curly or Wavy Hair: For curly or wavy hair, a layered cut will help to make your hairstyle look great. If you cut your hair blunt or too short, you hair will stand away or stick out from your head and face.

Haircut Tip: When you choose a specific haircut, the goal is to enhance your appearance in such a way that you look and feel beautiful. To ensure success, it is important to select hairstyles that enhance your facial shape. Descriptions of facial shapes and hairstyles that complement the shape or structure of the face follow. Find the shape that best matches yours.

Facial Structures

Oval

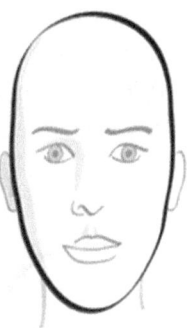

The oval shape face is the easiest facial structure to work with, as the proportions allow for virtually any hairstyle. To enhance the structure of an oval face, add layers that hang down the area of the cheekbones, lips, and chin to draw attention to your face. An oval face can wear bangs, and hair can be worn short or long, with styles such as a bob. If you are going out for the evening, wear your hair in an elegant upsweep or up-do style that is pulled back off the face, with or without wisps of hair hanging down. Your hairstyle options are essentially endless with this facial structure.

Square

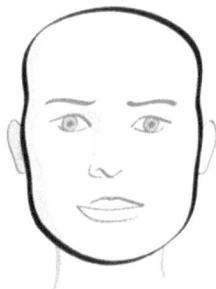

The square-shaped face has strong angles at the jaw and forehead. The hairstyle should allow for curves at the forehead with layered bangs that soften the look of the forehead. To accentuate this facial structure, begin layering the hair at the jawline. To soften the facial angles, allow some volume at the top of the head and sides (hair down with loose waves that frame the face). Avoid up-do styles, or use tendrils or wisps to soften the forehead and jawline. An off-center part breaks up symmetrical lines.

Round

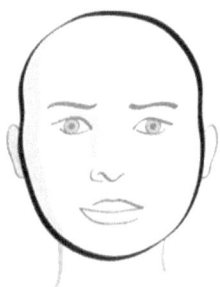

Most women consider the round-shaped face the least desirable, as it is usually associated with the appearance of weight gain. If your hair is thick on the sides, layer the sides of the hair and taper the hair below the chin level. Keeping the hair close to the side of the face, with low volume on top and long vertical lines, creates a longer facial appearance.

Rectangular

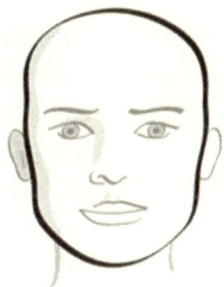

Rectangular is a common facial shape, easy to identify. It can appear angular or rounded. The hairstyle best suited to this facial shape has low volume at the top of the head and fullness on the sides of the face and helps to create the illusion of an oval shape.

Diamond

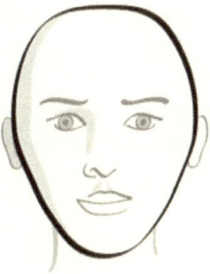

This shape is a cross between the oval and the heart-shaped face. It is widest at the cheekbones and narrow at the forehead and jawline. This facial shape lends itself to a multitude of hairstyles, but avoid wearing too much hair on your face, and choose hairstyles that add width to the chin area. Hairstyles with bangs will shorten the appearance of a long-looking face. Avoid too much hair on top and styles with hair near the chin area.

Tip: If you're not sure what facial-shape category you belong in, just remember these tips:

- Use soft curves and waves to minimize angles in the face shape.
- Use horizontal lines and curl to add width to a narrow area.
- Use vertical lines and lift to add height to a shortened or round face.
- Use styling elements (curved bangs, asymmetry, and off-center parting) to camouflage or distract from prominent features.

Using the right style elements will help you create the illusion of an oval-shaped face.

One-Length Haircut with Bangs

When cutting your hair, it is best to dampen the hair first, so keep a spray water bottle as part of your equipment arsenal. Dry hair has a tendency to fall into your eyes, making it difficult to see what you are doing. Allow an extra ¼ inch or more of length, as hair shrinks as it dries.

Equipment

    wall-mounted pull-out mirror
    spray bottle
    scissors
    comb

Cutting Instructions

To cut the front bang area, establish a guideline by cutting a small section in the middle of the bang.

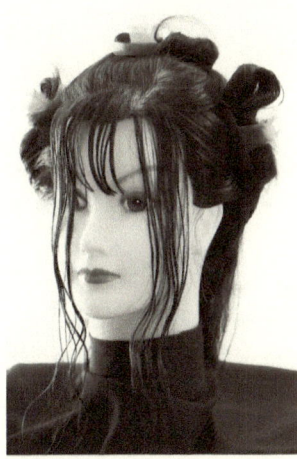

Do the same on the far end of each side of the bang. Now cut from the middle guideline to each side guideline. See how easy it is to get even bangs?

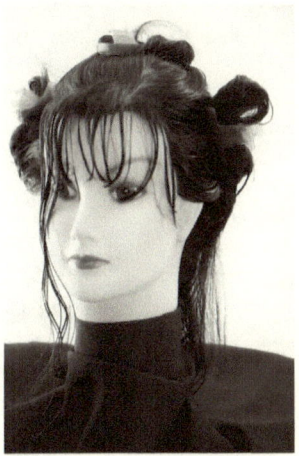

Cutting the Back and Sides of the Hair

To establish a cutting guideline at the back of the hair, looking at the back of your head in the wall-mounted pull-out mirror, cut a section of hair two to three inches from the center to the desired length.

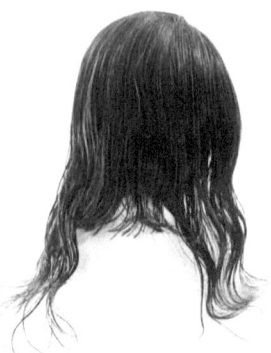

To establish a cutting guideline on each side of the head, cut from the back guideline up to the side guideline, and repeat the process on the opposite side of the head. Now slide your fingers down the remaining long section of hair to the side guideline, make sure it is even, and cut. Repeat this process on the other side of your head to complete the one-length haircut.

See the photo below, which shows how to establish back- and side-cutting guidelines.

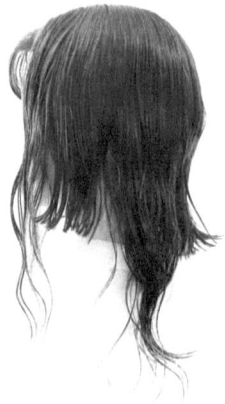

Finished one-length cut

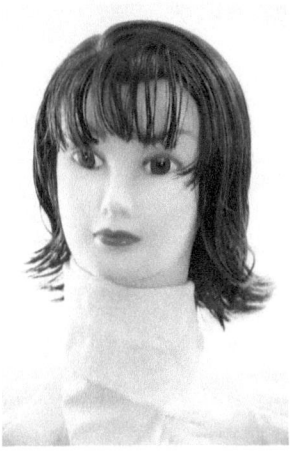

Layered Cut

With layered haircuts the shortest layer is the uppermost layer, with length increasing to the hair ends. Layered hairstyles rank among the most popular styles today. If your hair is long and straight, the layered look is a great choice. The layers also increase the appearance of volume, and color and highlighting add glitz and glamor to your hairstyle. The longer the hair, the more *visible* the layered hairstyle appears.

The layered hairstyle requires a *two-step* cutting process.

Step 1:

> Follow the instructions for a one-length cut to establish a guideline for the desired length. Part your hair into a rectangular section at the top of your head toward the front. Hold the hair upright at a ninety-degree angle between your index and middle fingers at the desired length. Starting at the front, using the shortest hair as a guide, cut toward the back of the hair you are holding between your fingers.

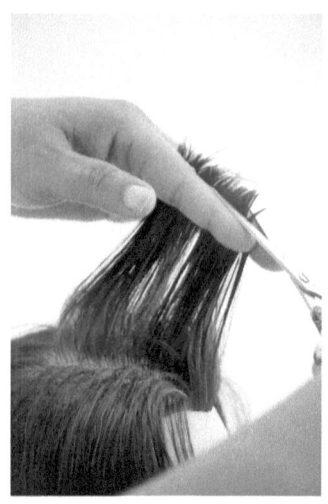

Step 2:

Now part your hair straight down the middle of your head (front to back). On the side of the part, make a two-inch section beginning in the front at the hairline, and clamp the remaining hair out of the way. Holding the hair at a ninety-degree angle, start to cut from the top guide, moving downward toward the bottom guideline. Continue the two-inch sectioning and clamping process until you reach the opposite side of the head.

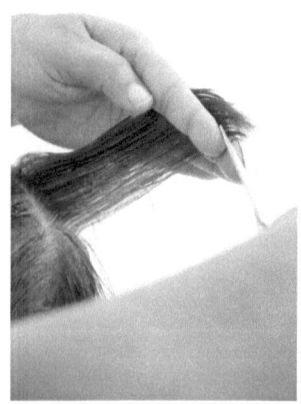

Finished Layered Cut

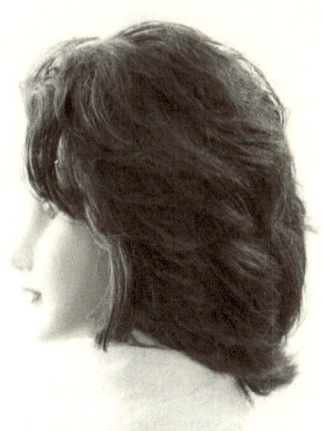

Tips for Clipper Cuts

Most clippers can be purchased as a complete set that includes cutting instructions. Some also have video instructions included. For best results, follow the instructions included. You can purchase larger attachments for longer cuts at your beauty supply store.

Basic Clipper-Cutting Instructions

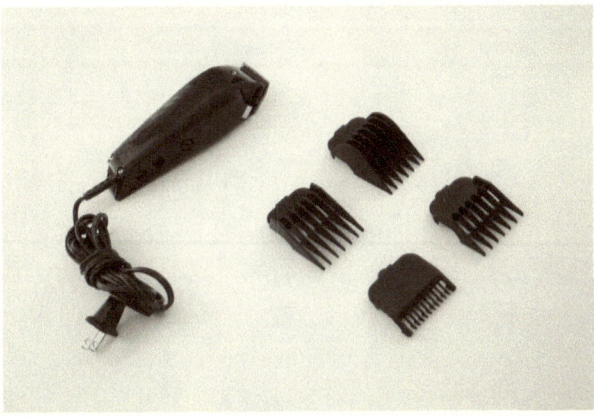

Take the clipper attachments out one at a time and slide them through the hair to see what size is required for the hairstyle you have selected. Be careful to select the correct size attachment:

Size 1 will be a cut close to the head.
Size 2 is an approximately ¼-inch cut.
Size 4 is an approximately ½-inch cut.
Size 6 is an approximately 1-inch cut.
Size 8 is an approximately 1¼-inch cut.

It is best to start the cut in the nape area, just above the neck, with the smallest attachment of your choice. If this is a man's haircut, you will use this same attachment to go around the ears. Select the next-highest attachment and continue clipping the hair evenly around the head. Then select the next-highest attachment and repeat until you are at the top of the head. Before you start cutting the top of the hair, select the attachment that will give you the length you desire and complete the cut on the remaining hair. Line up the nape area and the sides using a trimmer, not a clipper attachment, for this close cut or trim line to avoid nipping the skin.

CHAPTER 4

Tips on Hair Coloring

Hair color can enhance your looks, make you look radiant, and take years off your appearance. If you are going to color your or someone else's hair for the first time at home, be sure to keep the color selection simple by keeping it close to the hair's natural color.

Follow the instructions on the product information or instruction sheet closely and read all the information prior to starting the coloring process.

Types of Hair-Color Chemicals

Permanent color contains peroxide, so it does not wash out. You can expect this color to last four to six weeks before a retouch is needed.

To select the right permanent hair color, select a shade that is two to three shades lighter than or the same shade as your natural color. You can also choose a darker shade.

Semipermanent color, better known as temporary or shampoo-in color, does not contain peroxide. It can deposit color, but it will not lighten the hair. This type washes out in six to eight shampoos. The only options are to select your natural color or a darker shade.

Things to Consider

Consider the color of your skin when choosing hair color. Pale or pinkish skin tones are considered "cool" complexions. For this skin tone, use ash colors like wheat, champagne, or ash blond. If you have a cool complexion, avoid brassy tones like deep golds, reds, or auburn shades.

If your skin tone has a yellow, red, or olive tone, you have a "warm" complexion. Avoid ashy colors and choose auburns, caramel tones, golden browns, and blacks.

If you are applying color at home, you will not have a color chart at hand, so use the color on the box as your color guide.

For hair color and style variety, if you notice what you like in a magazine, cut the photo out and place it next to your face while looking in the mirror to evaluate whether the color and/or style looks good with your facial structure. The next step is to take the photo with you to the store to match the color with the color on the box.

Remember that color stains, so wear a protective plastic cape or old clothing, as it *will* get stained. Brush the hair away from your face, and place a petroleum-jelly product on your face by the hairline, on your ears, and around the nape of your neck to keep the color from staining your skin.

Dry, damaged hair tends to grab the hair color and be uneven, so make sure your hair is in good condition before applying color.

To remove hair color from the skin, put shampoo on a cotton ball or paper towel and apply it in a circular motion over the stain. You can also purchase color remover from a beauty supply store.

Note: Never use hair color if you have just had a perm or relaxed your hair. Wait seven to fourteen days, depending on the condition of your hair.

When washing your hair after applying a permanent hair color, make sure you shampoo the hair at least twice and rinse your hair completely until the rinse water is clear of color. Color left in the hair will cause hair damage.

Hair care done in the home can give to you the look you desire if you follow the manufacturer's instructions, examine the hair for healthiness, and apply the right conditioners and hair treatments as needed.

Color Retouching

When it's time for a touch-up of your color, apply the color to new hair growth only and allow the color to sit on the hair for twenty minutes. If there is any remaining color, add approximately one ounce of shampoo to the color, mix it, and then apply the mixture to the remaining hair. Comb through the hair with a large-tooth comb, allow the mixture to sit on the hair for ten minutes, shampoo twice, and rinse until the water is clear. Apply conditioner as directed and rinse. This process will brighten the hair while causing less damage from the coloring process.

Coloring Gray Hair

Gray hair may be resistant to hair coloring. If you have experienced difficulty covering the gray in your hair, you may want to purchase an additive from a beauty supply store to help the gray hair absorb the color. If you follow instructions closely, the additive will ensure maximum gray coverage, intensify and lock in the hair color, and promote longer color retention. The additive mixes with any permanent or semipermanent hair color. There are natural additives that include new technology that maximizes and ensures gray coverage. Always follow box instructions, and read the box label, as some hair colors will state "100 percent gray coverage."

Gray-Hair Challenges: Hair will appear gray when it loses color pigment. Gray hair can be resistant to color, so apply color to the gray hair first, and leave the color on the maximum amount of time. Sometimes gray hair will absorb too much red, purple, or green from the hair dye. If this happens (you have red or green hair and it's not Christmas), use the opposite base color. For example, if the hair is red or purple, choose an ash color, which has a green base. If the hair comes out green, choose golden browns or auburn to correct it.

Color-Neutral Protein Fillers

Protein fillers equalize hair porosity, allowing for even absorption of color. They restore and protect against hair damage from chemical processing and/or hot styling and assist in repairing damaged protein bonds. Color is sealed from the cortex, helping color last longer and giving hair volume and luster. The hair appears natural with even hair color, and it adjusts undesired ash tones that can be found in all shades of brown hair.

Hair Porosity

Porosity refers to the hair's ability to soak up moisture. If the hair is very porous, the hair cuticles are usually damaged, perhaps from overprocessing with bleaches, perms, or relaxers. Porous hair grabs and absorbs hair chemicals faster than nonporous hair and may become overprocessed and damaged quickly. Hair that is not very porous will not absorb chemicals quickly and may be difficult to perm or color.

To maintain beautiful, shiny colored hair, use shampoo and conditioning products made specifically for color-treated hair. These products have the necessary ingredients to condition and coat each hair strand, which preserves the hair color.

Highlighting at Home

Highlighting is very popular but can also be very expensive. You will be happy to know that there are highlighting kits that are designed to make it difficult to make a mistake with the application. These can be found at drug stores and beauty supply stores. To save a trip to the salon for correction, *do not ignore the instructions* that are included with the kit. Take the time to read and follow the instructions carefully. Some kits come with a cap with small holes and a hair hook that grabs the hair and you pull the hair through the holes, providing the hair is short enough to pull through.

If the hair is long, some kits come with an application wand, a brush, or control-touch applicators.

Low-Lighting at Home

If you have a bright hair color, such as sun-bleached or overhighlighted hair, and you want to tone it down, low-lighting kits are available for purchase in drug stores, retail stores, or online. When choosing a color for low-lighting, go one to two shades darker for a natural look.

If you have overhighlighted your hair and would like to tone the highlighted color down, you can. If your hair is in good condition, you should wait at least a week after highlighting before attempting the low-lighting. If the color of your hair requires immediate low-lighting, consult a professional colorist for correction.

Short Hair. You can purchase a cap and hook and the hair color (one to two shades darker) from a beauty supply store. After placing the cap tightly on your head, pull small strands of hair through the perforations in the cap and apply hair color to the exposed hair. (Follow the instructions closely when applying color.) After thirty minutes, rinse the color out before removing the cap. Remove the cap, and follow the shampooing instructions.

Longer Hair: You can purchase a bottle with an applicator made to apply color to the hair in even rows at a beauty supply or retail store or online. Mix the color in the applicator bottle, following the instructions included in the kit, and apply the mixture only to hair you would like to darken. If you have any doubts, make an appointment at your hair salon.

Important note: It is crucial that you read the packaged instructions in the coloring product. The allergy-testing instructions prior to product use could be lifesaving. If you have a tattoo, it may increase allergic reactions to coloring products. The allergy testing may need a forty-eight-hour window to allow for a potential reaction. Follow the instructions carefully!

Tips on Hair Perms

When shopping for a permanent wave to do at home, make sure you select the right product for your hair type, such as a perm for normal or for color-treated hair. There are two types of perms: alkaline and acid. Evaluate your hair texture and determine the best perm for you. Hair with low elasticity, highly resistant hair, coarse hair, and Asian hair types respond best to alkaline perms. Healthy hair, chemically treated hair, and weak hair types should be treated with a milder acid perm.

Make sure your hair is clean, and follow the directions completely, paying attention to the warnings and wrapping tips. Timing instructions are critical; if the permanent solution is left on the hair too long, it will cause significant damage by frying the hair, which you don't want to happen! Make sure your hair is wet before you start the rolling process with the perm rods, and do not allow the hair to dry before you apply the perm solution. Allow the appropriate amount of time for the perm solution to sit on the hair (ten to twenty minutes) before unwrapping one curl to determine whether this is the curl you want. If it is, rewrap the curl and rinse the hair (with the perm rods in) for approximately ten minutes. Towel-blot the hair dry with the rods still in, and apply neutralizer to each rod. Let the neutralizer sit for five minutes before removing the rods. Work the neutralizer through the hair with your fingers and then rinse the hair with cool water for five minutes. Finally, apply a leave-in conditioner. For best results, trim a quarter inch off the hair.

Do not shampoo for three days after a perm, and do not use a permanent hair color for seven to fourteen days. It is safe to use a semipermanent color after seventy-two hours.

Proper Placement of Perm Rods

When rolling the hair onto a perm rod, make sure that the rubber band on the perm rod is kept straight across when you snap it into place, or it will cause hair breakage after the perm. See the photo below for proper rod placement, and note the rubber-band placement.

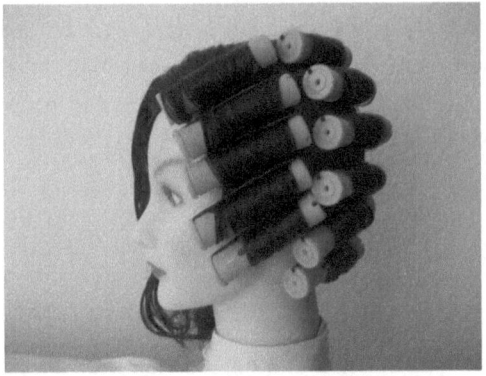

The size of the perm rod will determine the size of the curl. Small perm rods will result in tight curls, and large rods will make larger curls. All rods will produce a firm curl, and the curl will last the same amount of time, whether tight or large. A perm should last approximately three months with proper application and maintenance.

After seventy-two hours you can safely shampoo the hair and apply a deep conditioner for the health and appearance of your hair. If you shampoo and condition your hair before the seventy-two-hour mark, the perm may not last the expected amount of time.

When to Seek Professional Help

- If your hair is past shoulder length, go to a professional stylist for the perm because long hair may require a special wrapping technique to get the desired results.
- Extremely straight hair is difficult to wrap on the perm rod, so seek professional help for a professional perm that is designed for this hair type. You will be pleased in the end!
- Bleached hair that appears limp and damaged before the perm needs professional help, as the hair will sustain more damage with a home perm.
- Dry, brittle hair that has breakage will require a *weekly* deep conditioner for approximately four weeks *prior to applying any chemical* to avoid more damage to the hair.

Would you like to know what the style will look like before you do the perm? It's simple: Wet your hair, put the perm rods in your hair as if preparing to apply the chemical, allow the hair to dry, remove the rods, and comb the hair into the desired style. If you like it, proceed with the real perm.

A Reversed Permanent

If your hair is naturally curly and you want a straight hairstyle, or if you have a curly perm that is too curly, you can use the reverse perm method to straighten your hair.

Use a fine-tooth comb to work (comb) the perm solution through the hair until you see noticeable curl relaxation. At this point rinse the hair thoroughly until it is clear of the perm solution. Apply the neutralizer and comb it through hair. Wait five minutes. Rinse with cool water until the water is clear.

Tips on Hair Relaxing

When more control of the hair is needed for styling, some people relax their hair with a chemical relaxer. All chemical relaxers come with instructions, cautions, and warnings on the application process. For your hair's sake, don't ignore the instructions; they will direct you in the correct process, preserve your hair's health, and help you to achieve your goal of hair control and easier styling.

When shopping for relaxers, purchase a mild relaxer for thin hair, a regular relaxer for normal hair, or a super relaxer for thick, coarse hair.

After mixing the relaxer (follow directions for application), apply the relaxer to the hair using a chemical brush or the back of a comb. Apply a touch-up relaxer to new growth every six to nine weeks to avoid damage. Always have the hair tips cut after each relaxer, as the ends of the hair may be overprocessed and damaged, and trimming the ends will ensure a better style.

A deep-conditioning treatment is a good idea after each relaxer treatment, as the treatment will reach the center, or cortex, of the hair. Use of a hydrating leave-in conditioner after each shampoo will restore the hair moisture. Add a moderate amount of (oil-based) hair dressing to the hair; since relaxers tend to dry hair out, adding the hair dressing to the hair will help with moisture and improve control.

Temporary hair-straightener products are available at a beauty supply store. This product can be beneficial to use between relaxers or in place of a relaxer. Do not use a permanent hair color for seven to fourteen days after the relaxer has been applied. You can use a semipermanent color to limit damage to newly relaxed hair.

Humidity! Humidity! What Can I Do?

If you live in an area that has high humidity, keeping your relaxed hair looking silky may be difficult. Antihumidity products are available for purchase online and in beauty supply stores.

Managing Hair in a Humid Climate

The key to managing hair in a humid climate is to apply a moisturizer to your hair after every shampoo. During the summer, give your hair a vacation from flat irons and curling irons, which can dry and damage the hair, by wearing natural curls, letting your hair air-dry, or blow-drying on low to medium heat using a diffuser attachment. Overdrying will stress and damage your hair, causing it to frizz.

When Is It Safe to Straighten a Child's Hair?

To begin with, it is not necessary to straighten ethnic hair. All relaxer products contain chemicals that can cause damage to a child's developing scalp and hairline. Because of easy access to and the low cost of home relaxer kits made for children, we have the illusion that it is safe to use relaxers on children. However, children who have relaxer treatments may suffer permanent damage to their hair, including receding hairlines. It may be beneficial to consult a dermatologist regarding a safe age to start. In addition, because of the chemical base of relaxers, the child may experience stinging and/or burning of the scalp during the relaxer process. A temporary hair straightener may be an alternative until the child reaches an appropriate age at which it is safe to use a relaxer.

If you choose to relax your child's hair, have it done by a professional to ensure safe application and follow-through. In any case, relaxers are not recommended for use before age twelve.

CHAPTER 5

Common Causes of Hair Damage

The number-one cause of hair damage is *heat*. Heat from styling causes cuticles to crack and lose moisture, resulting in dry and brittle hair. It is important to use the recommended settings for each type of heating/ styling equipment to avoid hair damage.

Impact of Chemicals

Perms, relaxers, hair dye (especially with dye that contains peroxide), and bleaches cause damage to the hair cuticle, making it rough and increasing the chance that hair will break off.

Environmental Conditions: Your hair is exposed to the elements all year. Harsh weather conditions—winter cold, tropical heat, and direct sunlight—may cause your hair to become dry and brittle, resulting in breakage, particularly if it has been chemically processed. Why? There is less moisture in the air when it's cold, and the sun's UV rays break down hair protein.

Chemical Overlapping

Another cause of hair damage is chemical overlapping. When you have colored or permed hair, it is recommended that you apply any new relaxer or color only to new hair growth in the root area. When the chemical is applied to hair beyond the new growth, chemical overlapping causes damage with the additional application of the relaxer or color.

Overlapping time after time may cause the condition of the hair to break down, resulting in hair breakage.

Overprocessing with Chemicals

If your scalp begins to tingle, the relaxer has been left in too long, and the protective barrier you placed on your scalp is no longer working, causing possible temporary scalp damage. In addition, the hair is being broken down further.

Actual Experience

A single chemical process can damage the hair, so imagine what a "triple" chemical process can do. I once had a client who had applied a relaxer, hair color, and highlights at home, all within a few weeks, resulting in approximately 15–20 percent hair loss. I applied a protein deep conditioner and trimmed her hair into a style that limited the need for heat, which would cause more damage. We continued treatments for six weeks, and she changed her regular shampoo and conditioner to one for color-treated hair. We saw a marked improvement in a few short weeks. My client realized that deep conditioning is a must when using chemicals and understood the importance of protecting the hair and using heat-protecting products.

www.ingramcontent.com/pod-product-compliance
Lightning Source LLC
Chambersburg PA
CBHW050337290526
45785CB00006B/2536